Group-Based Interventions for Coping with Brain Injury for Families

This combined manual and workbook allows clinicians to develop and run an 'Understanding Brain Injury' group-based intervention for the families of patients who have suffered moderate to severe brain injury. This is a specific group-based course useful for family groups with patients who are in hospital or early discharge. Taking an approach based on psycho-education and cognitive behaviour therapy, the manual guides the facilitator through each session, outlining what should be focused on, giving suggestions for talking points, and enabling the group to become a lively, interactive unit in which the members share their own experiences and gain insight and caregiving coping strategies from each other.

The manual is accompanied by a full workbook, available as an appendix and also in downloadable format in an accompanying eResource. After working through the programme, the families of the individual with the brain injury will have a better understanding of the consequences of their family member's condition, and be helped to devise personalised solutions for these difficulties. The workbook also includes an overview of the brain and explains how damage to different areas can have physical, cognitive, behavioural, emotional, and lifestyle consequences.

This manual and workbook will be invaluable to a range of health and social care professionals and trainees working with those with brain injury in group settings.

Rebekah Jamieson-Craig is a senior clinical psychologist specialising in neuropsychology, with 15 years of experience in working with adults who have acquired brain injuries, in both inpatient post-acute settings and slow-stream rehabilitation units. She has developed and run the 'Understanding Brain Injury' group extensively over this period.

Group-Based Interventions for Coping with Brain Injury for Families

A Manual and Workbook for Practitioners and Family Caregivers

Rebekah Jamieson-Craig

Routledge
Taylor & Francis Group
LONDON AND NEW YORK

Designed cover image: Getty Images

First published 2026
by Routledge
4 Park Square, Milton Park, Abingdon, Oxon OX14 4RN

and by Routledge
605 Third Avenue, New York, NY 10158

Routledge is an imprint of the Taylor & Francis Group, an informa business

British Library Cataloguing-in-Publication Data
A catalogue record for this book is available from the British Library

ISBN: 978-1-041-15526-3 (hbk)
ISBN: 978-1-041-15521-8 (pbk)
ISBN: 978-1-003-67988-2 (ebk)

DOI: 10.4324/9781003679882

Typeset in Optima
by Apex CoVantage, LLC

Access the support material: www.routledge.com/9781041155263

Contents

Acknowledgements

With thanks to Dr Tarick Ali, clinical psychologist, who helped me conceptualise how to create the 'Understanding Brain Injury' groups.

Also, thanks to the many trainee clinical psychologists and assistant psychologists, without whom the group would not have run as successfully for so many years.

1 Why Create this Manual?

This manual has been created to help anyone who wishes to run an Understanding Brain Injury group for family members who have been affected by brain injury. It is to be used in conjunction with the Understanding Brain Injury information pack. The group is to be an interactive group, in which all the members tell their own stories and describe the difficulties they are experiencing since their loved one had the brain injury.

The idea for this group stemmed from the original 'Understanding Brain Injury' group, which was created to help individuals coping with the effects of brain injury. In this group, different aspects of how a brain injury affects a person's life are discussed, alongside how this affects them emotionally. Finally, coping strategies are considered in a solution-focused manner. This group has not only successfully run for many years in a variety of settings, but the manual and workbook that resulted have also been published. At the time of devising the 'Understanding Brain Injury' group it was acknowledged that family members would benefit from a space where they could discuss the emotional effects of the brain injury on their own wellbeing, as well as develop coping skills to manage both the challenges that the brain injury produces and on their own mental wellbeing.

Over the years, groups have been devised for family members or loved ones following a brain injury, but many of these focus on education about the brain injury and on how to help the survivor continue with their lives despite the challenges of the brain injury. They are often skills-building or psychoeducational in nature (Kreutzer et al., 2015; Backhaus et al., 2010). Although there are components of this in this group, the fundamental

DOI: 10.4324/9781003679882-1

difference is that the current manual emphasises discussing how the loved one is coping with the changes to their own lives, rather than predominantly considering the changes that the individual with brain injury is living with.

Feedback from past participants on what they found valuable about attending a group includes statements such as: 'Hearing people going through the same thing as I am going through, makes it normal', 'You think you are the only one and feel guilty; it made me realise lots of people feel similar things and that was really helpful', 'I feel less isolated now I know it's not just me that feels this way', 'It was very helpful to see that I am not alone in this', and 'It's good to hear how others are coping, then I can try their strategies myself'. I have found that keeping the structure of a group relatively loose, so that the individuals can speak freely about what they are struggling with, is really important. The group hopefully helps participants acknowledge the complexity of living with a loved one who has a brain injury and, in doing so, it will aid in the building of coping strategies that many may find useful. After a brain injury occurs, there will be several challenges for any loved one, from getting used to using mobility aids or receiving help with communication to learning to live with emotional, behavioural, and personality changes that may occur. There is no one-size-fits-all approach to working either with the individual with brain injury or with their close others; rather, a case-by-case approach is more appropriate. In this sense, I cannot tell you what each group will find the most useful in any session, as each person will come with their own strengths and challenges and will perceive the brain injury differently. Some may struggle to accept what has happened, especially emotionally, while others may be more robust emotionally but be looking for practical coping skills to manage the everyday challenges of caring for someone with a brain injury. Each group, in my experience, will be different.

This group comprises four sessions. In this manual I will go through each one individually outlining what can be done and giving ideas for questions that can be asked of the group to elicit discussion about their difficulties and what coping strategies they have encountered and found helpful.

References

Backhaus, S. L., Ibarra, S. L., Klyce, D., Trexler, L. E., & Malec, J. F. (2010). Brain injury coping skills group: A preventative intervention for patients with brain injury and their caregivers. *Archives of Physical Medicine and Rehabilitation*, *91*(6), 840–848.

Kreutzer, J. S., Marwitz, J. H., Sima, A. P., & Godwin, E. E. (2015). Efficacy of the brain injury family intervention: Impact on family members. *The Journal of Head Trauma Rehabilitation*, *30*(4), 249–260.

2 Introducing the Group

Understanding Brain Injury group for families (or loved ones), or UBIF for short, is a group designed to increase the family members' insight into the cause and effects of the brain injury, help them identify the changes and difficulties the injured person is experiencing since their brain injury, and what they can do to help cope with these changes. This group is just as much about giving the individuals space to discover that they are not alone in having family members who suffer from a brain injury, to learn from each other's experiences, as it is to discover new ways of coping with the challenges of surviving a brain injury.

Each group itself holds four sessions, each of which will be covered in the following chapters. Before starting the group, however, certain factors should be considered. For example, how many facilitators are needed to run the group? What size should the group be? How long should each session be? What about the group mix – gender, age, loved one's disability? Are there any reasons to exclude someone from the group? Should the group be closed or open to new attendees each week? Each of these questions is valid, and although I cannot tell you what would definitively be best, I can tell you what I think will help when running this group.

Facilitators

Even though it is possible to run this group on your own, it is helpful if there are two people to co-facilitate. Generally, one person would lead the group asking the questions and importing information where appropriate, while the other person aids by writing the suggestions made by the group on the

DOI: 10.4324/9781003679882-2

flipchart. Often, my co-facilitator and I would switch roles each session so that the group could benefit from the slightly different styles each person has when running a group.

Size

The ideal number of participants is up to ten. It can be quite difficult to facilitate a group and make sure that all the members are getting a chance to get their point across. With smaller groups, it is more feasible for everyone who wishes to speak to be given ample space and time to do so. Another consideration to be made regarding group size is that smaller groups can then take place in more relaxed settings.

Length

It is best to give 1 to 1.5 hours to complete each UBIF session. It can be useful to have a little extra time when doing the sessions specifically looking at the difficulties caused by brain injury, as often group members will become quite involved in discussing what they are finding challenging. A further point is the frequency of the group. Again, this is up to the facilitator, but I found it helpful to run one session a week, or possibly fortnightly – this way the group was easier to fit in around the participants' already busy lives.

Group mix

The heterogeneity of the group can be both a benefit and a pitfall. I have run groups in brain injury units where the family members have experienced a wide range of brain injuries, but I have also run this group for specific conditions, such as stroke. Both have been successful and both pose their own challenges. It helps to have knowledge of the brain injury that a loved one has had and how it has affected them. This way, you can try to mitigate some of the difficulties that might arise when running a group with participants whose lived experiences differ. With regard to whether there are reasons to exclude people from the group, the only issue that I have found difficulty with is language – for example, if a participant has little or no English (or whatever the predominant language being spoken is), then they will have difficulty joining in with the group.

Another area for consideration is whether the group should be an open or closed group. There are benefits to both of these types of groups, but I have found that keeping the participants the same throughout the four sessions is usually best, as that way the group can become more cohesive, and trust and understanding can be built between the members. A lack of consistency in the group members can, at times, hinder the flow, especially if members do not know each other or what was spoken about in the previous group session.

Before the start of the first session, there are a few other things that must be considered. First, where will the group session take place? Personally, I found it most beneficial to run the group in a small room where all the members could sit around one table. This seemed to increase the group's cohesiveness. Second, it helps if there are blank walls in the room so that as the group progresses the previous week's information can be stuck up as an *aide memoire*. This way the group rules are accessible to all the members throughout. This leads me nicely to the idea of using a flipchart. By using a flipchart and different coloured pens, the group's ideas can be recorded as the members suggest them. It can also be used to help explain some of the more complex ideas, such as the functions of the different lobes of the brain. With this in mind, I found it incredibly useful to have a plastic model brain that depicted the different lobes as well as the two hemispheres.

In the post-pandemic world we now live in, people have become accustomed to the use of video-conferencing software. I have run groups using this format, and although they have their own challenges, they can often be easier for the family members as they do not need to leave their loved ones or homes to attend. When using video-conferencing, the same suggestions apply – use a whiteboard or flipchart positioned so that everyone can see it, and share the facilitation as before. If you have the software, PowerPoint or Whiteboard functions on video-conferencing programs could be used rather than the pen-and-paper flipcharts. Photos of the completed flipchart (or PowerPoint/Whiteboard functions) can be taken and shared with the group via email at the end of each session.

3 Session 1 What Is the Understanding Brain Injury Group?

Before the group begins, make sure you are aware of what has happened to each of the group members' loved ones. This means not only what type of brain injury they have sustained, but also when it occurred and which hospital they were taken to – additionally, try to discover any information on their family, previous jobs and hobbies .

For this session, a plastic model brain is really helpful. Also, multi-coloured pens can help illustrate what the different lobes of the brain do.

At the start of the group, it is useful to have the name of the group and the title of the session written on the flipchart. For the group to work well, all members need to be introduced not only to one another but also to the idea that they are going to learn about brain injury and the effects it can have on their lives as well as on their loved ones' lives. This may well be the first time many members of the group have met each other. With this in mind, it is useful to get all of the members to give their names and tell the group something about their loved one. Write the members' names on a sheet of the flipchart so that it can be stuck on the walls for future sessions. Add to this sheet the names of the co-facilitators.

Move on to explain how there will be four sessions and outline briefly what each of these sessions will comprise.

Next, it is time for the group to decide on some 'group rules'. It is best if the members are asked to come up with their own rules that they would like everyone to follow within the group; however, if they struggle to produce their own list, there are suggestions in the information pack. Write on the flip-chart all the rules the group members agree on so that they can be referred to later if necessary. Typically, this will include confidentiality. Although this is important, it should be emphasised that, if any sort of risk is mentioned, then

DOI: 10.4324/9781003679882-3

this will need to be brought to the wider team to ensure the group member, their family, and the individual with the brain injury remain safe.[1]

After the rules have been agreed upon, go on to discuss the prevalence of brain injury within the UK and abroad. This section can be quite powerful; frequently, the family members will be surprised to find out how common brain injury is and how many people are living with the long-term effects of brain injury in the United Kingdom alone. Statements such as 'so we're not alone', 'I never realised so many people continued life with a brain injury', 'I thought it was really uncommon . . . just us . . . I don't know anyone else with a brain injury ' are frequently made after this section of the session. This, I think, starts to help some members feel less isolated and alone.

Following this, the session is then divided into three separate sections.

The **first section** highlights what our brains do. It starts by describing the two hemispheres and explaining what general functions each of the hemispheres is responsible for. This can be found in the information pack as well as in Appendix 1 of this manual. It can be useful to write these up on the flipchart as you describe them. Following this, the areas of the brain are explored. To help with this, the model brain should be handed around and the different lobes pointed out. It can also help to point to where the lobes are on your own head. Within the information pack are very basic descriptions of the function of each of the lobes, however, in the group session it can help to go into slightly more detail. As you describe what each lobe does, it is really helpful to draw a diagram of the brain, label the lobes, and note down the most salient parts of what each lobe does. To help you with this information a list has been provided in Appendix 1 of this manual.

The **second section** of this session focuses on different causes of brain injury. Within the information pack are the most common causes of brain injury; however, it may be necessary for you to talk about more obscure forms of brain injury if a group member's loved one has acquired this. Generally, though, most forms will be covered by the primary five types that are in the pack: stroke (this includes haemorrhages), hypoxia (heart attack, poisoning, anaphylaxis, electrocution), traumatic (falls, road traffic accidents [RTAs], assaults), tumours, and infections.

Finally, in the **third section**, the group members are encouraged to think about what changes their loved one has experienced since their brain injury. These can be broken down into changes that can be seen (physical) and changes that cannot be seen (mental). This can be structured as a table with two columns on the flipchart for the members to fill in as a group.

Session 1 in summary

- Items needed for this session include a flipchart, coloured markers, and copies of the information pack for each participant. If conducting the group virtually, I suggest emailing the information pack to the participants the day before.
- Get to know your participants before the group starts. What happened to their loved one? When? Where were they treated? Previous jobs, hobbies etc.
- Write the name of the group and title of the session on the flipchart.
- Introduce members to the group, to one another and to yourselves.
- Ask whether there is anything in particular the members would like to discover about their loved ones' brain injuries
- Discuss group rules. Write these on the flipchart.
- Discuss the prevalence of brain injury in the UK.
- Describe our brains, i.e. the two hemispheres, the different lobes and their functions. Use the plastic model brain to help illustrate the lobes.
- Draw a diagram of the brain, label the lobes, and note down the most salient functions of each.
- Discuss the different causes of brain injury and help the group members identify which of these causes apply to their loved one.
- Encourage the group members to think about what changes they have experienced since their loved ones experienced the brain injury (physical, mental). Share these as a group and write them up on the flipchart.
- Recap what has been learned today.

Note

1 It is possible that a member of the group may disclose a wish to harm either themself or the individual with the brain injury, or they may indicate a concern about being harmed by the person with the brain injury. If any of these were to be the case, then it would be unethical to keep them entirely confidential. Rather, such concerns would need to be taken to the wider team and would also need to be discussed with the person on a one-to-one basis, possibly even contacting their GP or social services depending on the level of risk being disclosed

4 Session 2
Physical Changes After Brain Injury

The purpose of this session is three-fold. First, to increase the group members' understanding of the physical effects of the brain injury on their loved ones. Second, to increase their awareness of the impact of the brain injury on their own coping strategies. And third, to help the members identify sources of support that are available to them.

On the flipchart, write '**Physical changes**' in the centre. Ask the members of the group what physical changes they have noticed within their loved ones, as well as within other people who have experienced brain injury. Note these down on the flipchart in a spider diagram format (see Appendix 3). Once the group members have exhausted their list, check in the information pack, see if there are any further difficulties listed in the information pack that the group identify with (see Appendix 2 for a more expansive list of physical changes). Ask the group what physical changes they have noticed within themselves that have occurred due to their loved ones' brain injuries.

Next, ask the group members what the emotional consequences of their loved ones having these physical changes are for them. Write these responses in a different colour radiating out from the changes. Again, prompt questions might be necessary to get the members really thinking about how they feel – for example, when they cannot do something they used to do, without it being considerably more difficult. Examples of these questions could be: When you realise you can no longer do X because of your loved one's disability, how does that make you feel? What does it make you think of yourself? These emotions do not have to directly correlate to any one difficulty; rather, they are emotions that may or may not be elicited by any of the difficulties mentioned. Again, once the group think they have mentioned all the

DOI: 10.4324/9781003679882-4

emotions that having these changes elicits from them, check the information pack to see if there is anything that has been forgotten.

Following this, the next area of discussion should be to do with coping strategies. For this, an additional three coloured pens should be used: one colour to signify problem-based strategies; one colour for emotion-based strategies; and a further colour for distraction-based strategies. These should be written on the spider diagram, radiating out from the emotions. These can often be quite difficult to elucidate from the group as the members may not feel they are coping. Questions that may help in this situation are: 'What do you do to distract yourself from these thoughts and feelings?', 'How do you deal with these difficulties on a daily basis?'. As with the list of emotions, each coping strategy does not have to correspond directly to one emotion; rather, this is just a visual representation depicting the fact that there may be many different coping strategies that can help with the emotions and difficulties that occur after brain injury. Once more, when the group members think they have given a full account of all the strategies they use to help them cope with both the difficulties and the feelings the physical changes have caused, check in the information pack to see if any more should be included, as there is a page dedicated to this.

Finally, at the bottom of the flipchart sheet, a list of suggestions of who the members can turn to for help and advice should be written down in yet another colour. This list should come from the members as much as possible.

See Appendix 3 for an example of the '**Physical changes**' spider diagram.

Session 2 in summary

- Items that will be needed for this session include the flipchart and coloured marker pens.
- Write the name of the group and title of the session on the flipchart.
- Recap the first session.
- On the flipchart write '**Physical changes**' in the centre.
- Ask the members of the group what physical changes they have noticed within their loved ones and in other people who have experienced brain injury as well as within themselves.
- Note these down on the flipchart, radiating from the central '**Physical changes**' title.

- Check the information pack to see whether there are any further changes the group has not generated but would identify with. Add these to the flipchart.
- Ask the group members what the emotional consequences of their loved ones having these changes are for themselves. Write their responses in a different colour, radiating out from the changes.
- Once the group think they have mentioned all of the emotions that these changes elicit from them, check the information pack to see if anything has been forgotten.
- Ask the group for suggestions on how they have coped with these emotions. Use a different colour pen depending on whether the suggestion is problem-based, emotion-based, or distraction-based. Write these coping strategies down radiating out from the emotions.
- Once the group thinks they have mentioned all the strategies they use to help them cope with both the difficulties and the feelings the physical changes have caused, check with the information pack.
- Suggestions of who the members can turn to for help and advice should be written down in yet another colour at the bottom of the flipchart.
- Make a note of the different colours used on this flipchart so you can apply the same colours to similar categories in the later flipcharts.

5 Session 3 Mental Process Changes After Brain Injury

Again, as with Session 2, there are three main objectives to this session: to increase the members' understanding of the effects of the brain injury on their loved ones' mental processes (thinking skills, emotions, behaviours); second, to increase their awareness of the impact of the brain injury on their own coping strategies; and third, to help the members identify sources of support that are available to them.

As usual, start the session by going back to the spider diagram that was created in the last session and refreshing the group's memory of what was discussed. It can be really useful to stick this spider diagram up on the wall so that the members can refer to it throughout the rest of the sessions.

This time write '**Mental process changes**' in the centre of the flipchart. As with the session on physical changes, try to get the group members to generate as many mental process changes as they can independently. These include changes in thinking (memory, planning, problem-solving, speed of thinking, etc.), emotions (becoming sad, anxious, stressed, etc.), and behaviour (losing temper more easily, lack of social skills, etc.), and write them down emanating from the central '**Mental process changes**'. Unlike with physical changes, these can be more difficult for the group to produce as these changes are not always so obvious (see Appendix 4 for a comprehensive list). Once the group members have exhausted their list, check in the information pack and see if there are any further difficulties listed there that the group might identify with.

Following this, ask the group what emotions these changes in their loved ones elicit from them. Write these on the flipchart in a separate colour, spreading out from the list of changes. As with the feelings about physical changes, it is likely that prompt questions will be needed to encourage the

DOI: 10.4324/9781003679882-5

group members to think about how they are feeling about their loved ones' mental process difficulties. Similarly to the physical changes, these emotions do not have to directly correlate to any one difficulty; rather they are emotions that may or may not be elicited by any of the difficulties mentioned. Once the group think they have mentioned all the ways these difficulties make them feel, check in the information pack to see whether there are any further emotions that the group recognise.

Next, ask the group to generate a list of coping strategies that help them with both the difficulties as well as the feelings they have in relation to these difficulties. Again, as with the physical changes, these coping strategies should be written in differing coloured pens, depending on whether they are problem-based, emotion-based, or distraction-based. The colour of the pen should be the same as the one used when discussing coping strategies for physical changes. Write these on the flipchart, radiating from the feelings about '**Mental process changes**' as a visual representation of strategies that can assist with the difficulties and the emotions these changes cause. Once more, when the group think they have given a full account of all the strategies they use to help them cope with both the difficulties and the feelings the changes have caused within them, check in the information pack as there is a page dedicated to this.

Finally, at the bottom of the flipchart sheet, suggestions of people whom the members can turn to for help and advice should be generated by the group and written down in yet another colour.

See Appendix 5 for an example of the '**Mental process changes**' spider diagram.

Session 3 in summary

- Items that will be needed for this session include the flipchart and coloured markers. For the different categories below, use the same colours as used for the 'Physical changes' flipchart.
- Write the name of the group and title of the session on the flipchart.
- Recap the second session.
- On the flipchart write '**Mental process changes**' in the centre.
- Try to get the group members to generate as many mental process changes as possible that they have noticed within their loved ones.

- Note these down on the flipchart, radiating from the central '**Mental process changes**' title.
- Check the information pack to see whether there are any further changes the group has not generated but would identify with. Add these to the flipchart.
- Ask the group what emotions these changes elicit within them. Write their responses in a different colour, radiating from the changes.
- Ask the group members for suggestions of coping strategies that have helped them with these difficulties and emotions. Write these coping strategies down radiating from the emotions in different colour pens.
- Once the group members think they have mentioned all the strategies they use to help them cope with both the difficulties and the feelings the changes have caused, check with the information pack.
- Suggestions of who the members can turn to for help and advice should be generated and written down in yet another colour at the bottom of the flipchart.
- Recap what has been learned in the session.

6 Session 4
Lifestyle Changes After Brain Injury

This is the last session and it will be based on using the spider diagram format. As with the previous two sessions, its emphasis is on trying to encourage each member to identify the changes to their lifestyle caused by their loved one's brain injury. The aim for this session is to help the members understand how their own lifestyles have been affected, aiding them in recognising the feelings they have about these changes, and finally facilitating their discovery of coping strategies for both the changes and the emotions they feel regarding these differences.

On a new sheet of the flipchart write '**Lifestyle changes**'. Ask each member of the group what changes they have experienced in their lifestyle since their loved one had the brain injury. Write all the changes that the group produce on the flipchart, radiating from the central '**Lifestyle changes**'. A list of lifestyle changes has been incorporated in Appendix 6 to help.

From here, as with the previous sessions, feelings about these lifestyle changes need to be addressed. Enquire what emotions the members feel when thinking about the lifestyle changes they have had to deal with or are expecting to need to deal with in the future. Write this list of feelings on the spider diagram, spreading out from the changes. As with the other diagrams, the emotions do not need to directly correlate to a specific change.

Next, ask the group members what coping strategies they use to help them with the changes to their lifestyles as well as with the emotions that these changes cause. Again, these coping strategies should be grouped by colour pen, depending on whether they are problem-based, emotion-based, or distraction-based. Continue to use the same colour pens as were used in 'Mental process changes' and 'Physical changes'. This section is particularly important as it is looking at how the members are going to cope with their

DOI: 10.4324/9781003679882-6

lifestyle changes in the future. Write down all suggestions on the flipchart, emanating from the emotions, as with the other spider diagrams.

As with the other sessions, a list of people who the members can turn to for advice and support with their lifestyle changes should be generated and written down in a different colour.

See Appendix 7 for an example of the '**Lifestyle changes**' spider diagram.

As this is the final session, thank the participants and answer any further questions the group may have generated.

In my experience, some group members might wish to keep in contact with each other, I have offered to send out email addresses to those I have mutual consent from.

After the group has ended, create copies of the spider diagrams for all three coping skills sessions and send these to the participants, either via email or post, so that they have a copy of what was discussed throughout the group.

Session 4 in summary

- Items that will be needed for this session include the flipchart and coloured markers. For the different categories below, use the same colours as used for the ''Physical changes' flipchart.
- Write the name of the group and title of the session on the flipchart.
- Recap the third session.
- On the flipchart write '**Lifestyle changes**' in the centre.
- Try to get the group to generate as many lifestyle changes as possible that they have noticed within their own lives.
- Note these down on the flipchart, radiating from the central '**Lifestyle changes**' title.
- Check the information pack to see whether there are any further changes the group have not generated but would identify with. Add these to the flipchart.
- Ask the group what these changes make them feel about themselves and their lives. Write their responses in a different colour, radiating from the changes.
- Once the group think they have mentioned all the emotions that these changes elicit from them, check the information pack to see if anything has been forgotten.

- Ask the group for suggestions of things that have helped them with these difficulties and the way they feel about themselves. Write these coping strategies down, grouping by using different coloured pens depending on whether they are problem-based, emotion-based, or distraction-based, radiating out from the emotions.
- Once the group members think they have mentioned all the strategies they use to help them cope with both the difficulties and the feelings the lifestyle changes have caused, check with the information pack.
- Suggestions of who the members can turn to for help and advice should be generated and written down in yet another colour at the bottom of the flipchart.
- Recap what has been learned in the session.
- Find out whether group members wish to remain in contact, and those who do, get consent to share email addresses.

Appendix

1 Areas of the Brain

Right hemisphere: Controls the left side of the body.

Creative aspects: responsible for rhythm, spatial awareness, colour, imagination, daydreaming, holistic awareness, dimension.

Left hemisphere: Controls the right side of the body.

Logical brain: responsible for words, logic, numbers, analysis, lists, linearity, and sequencing.

Frontal lobe: Positioned at the foremost region of the cerebral cortex.

Involved in: motor functions, decision-making, planning, problem-solving, reasoning, judgement, impulse control, personality, attention, organisational abilities, motivation, regulation of emotions.

Parietal lobe: Positioned towards the top and back of the cerebral cortex.

Involved in: integrating sensory information from various parts of the body, knowledge of numbers and their relationships, manipulation of objects, processing information related to touch, visuospatial processing.

Temporal lobe: Positioned to the side of the cerebral cortex.

Involved in: auditory perception, memory, speech, comprehension, emotional responses, visual perception.

Occipital lobe: Positioned at the back of the cerebral cortex.

Involved in: visual processing.

Appendix

2

Physical Changes

Difficulties with:

- Sitting
- Balance
- Standing
- Walking
- Weakness
- Movement
- Tiredness
- Fatigue
- Pain
- Using arm/hand
- Vision
- Hearing
- Muscle tension
- Muscle tone
- Coordination
- Swallowing
- Dizziness
- Speech
- Appetite change
- Loss of sensation
- Incontinence
- Epilepsy

Changes within the group members:

- Increased tiredness
- Sleep difficulties
- Inability to exercise
- Changes in appetite

Appendix 3

Example Spider Diagram of Physical Changes

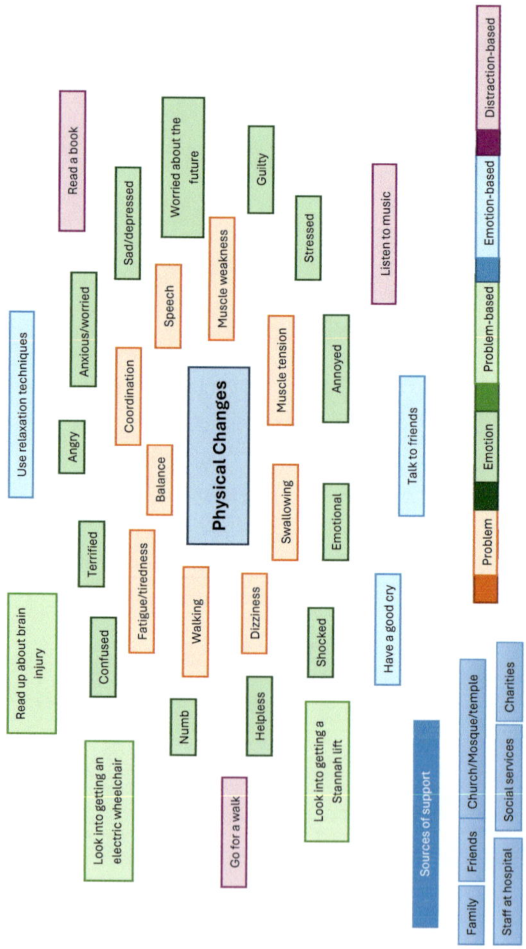

Appendix

4 Mental Process Changes

Difficulties with:

- Memory – short- and long-term
- Retrograde amnesia
- Anterograde amnesia
- Planning
- Problem-solving
- Decision-making
- Organising
- Reasoning
- Attention
- Concentration
- Speed of information processing
- Visuospatial abilities
- Perceptual abilities
- Speaking
- Reading
- Writing
- Confusion
- Disorientation
- Understanding
- Impulsivity
- Impatience
- Anger
- Sadness

- Anxiety/worry
- Sexual urges
- Social skills

Changes within the group members:

- Increased fatigue
- Difficulty concentrating
- Feeling overwhelmed

Appendix

5

Example Spider Diagram of Mental Process Changes

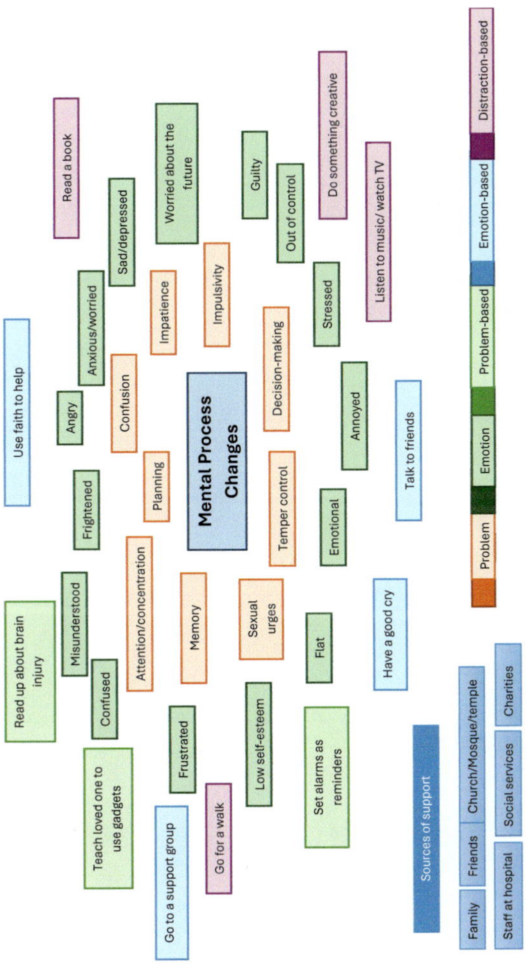

Appendix

6 Lifestyle Changes

Difficulties with:

- Daily activities
    - Showering
    - Dressing
    - Toileting
- Cooking
- Shopping
- Housing
- Driving
- Travelling
- Family roles
- Relationships
- Friendships

Changes for the group members:

- Financial worries
- Change in life roles
- Change in intimacy

Appendix

7

Example Spider Diagram of Lifestyle Changes

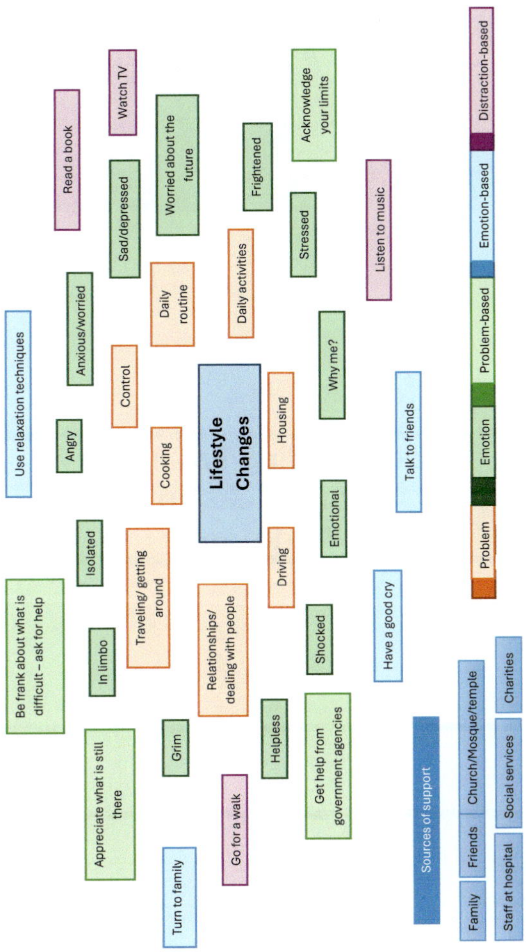

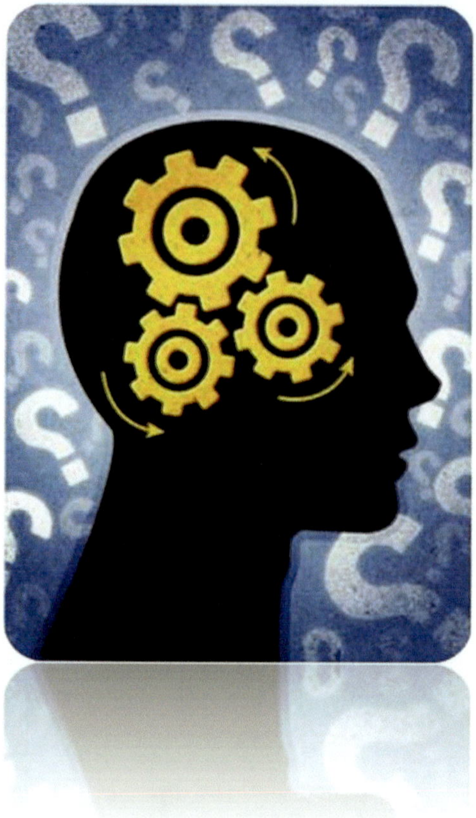

Understanding Brain Injury Family Group Workbook

Date:

Name:

Introduction	
	This group is about:
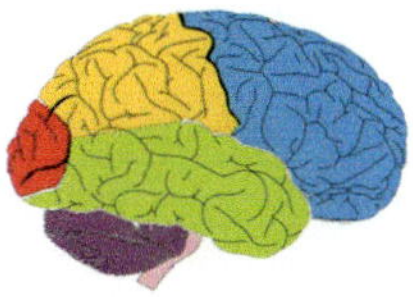	• Learning more about the brain
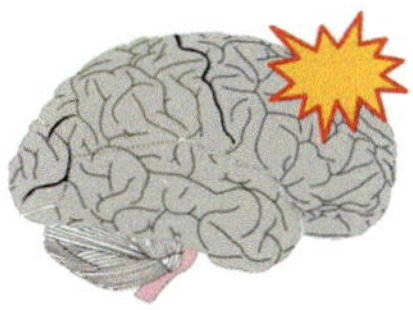	• Understanding what brain injury is
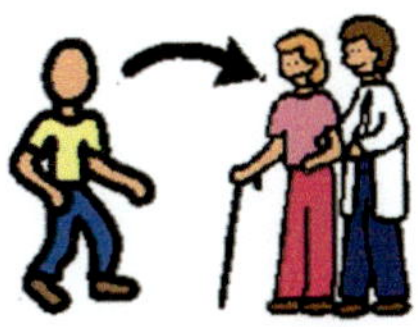	• Learning about the effects of brain injury and how these have impacted your lives
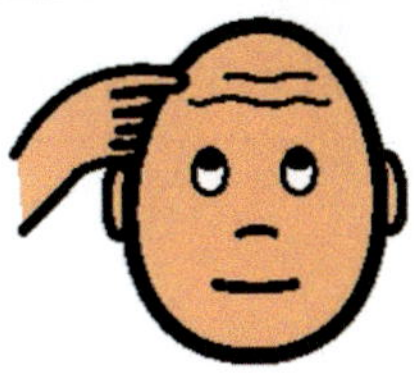	• Thinking about what you can do to cope with these changes to your loved one and to your own life

	Contents
	There are **four** group sessions:
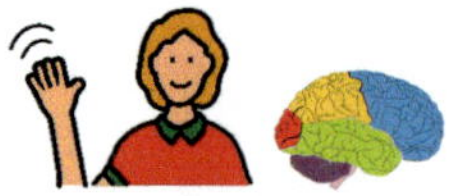	1. Introduction, the brain and brain injury
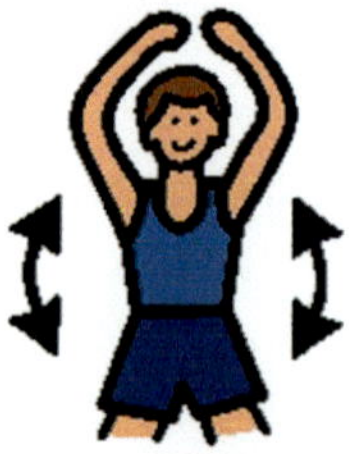	2. Physical changes after brain injury
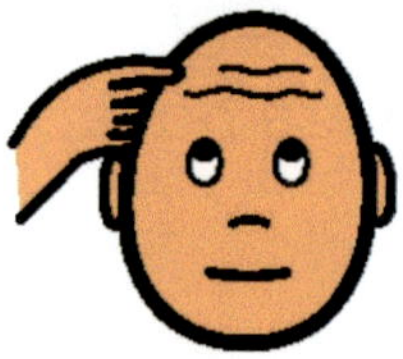	3. Mental process changes after brain injury
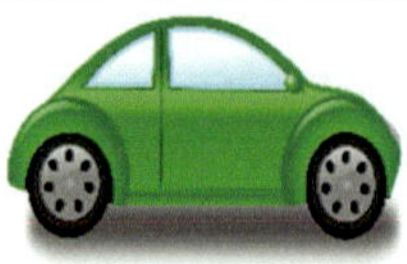	4. Lifestyle changes after brain injury

Session 1

Introduction to the Understanding Brain Injury Group

	In this session, we will:	
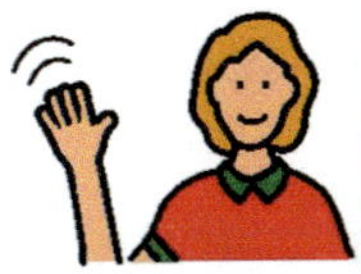		Introduce the group members
		Make some group rules
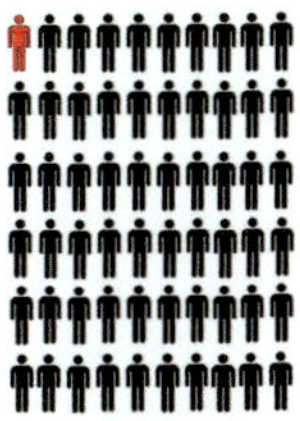		Find out how common brain injury is
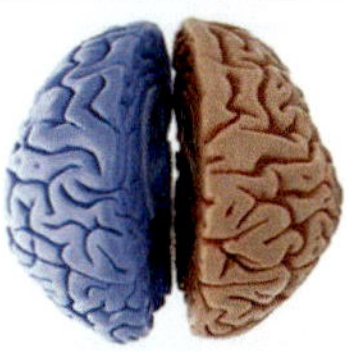		The brain
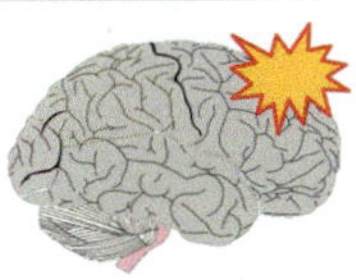		Types of brain injury

Group Rules

Here are some suggested group rules:

- Be on time
- Let everyone have the same time to speak
- Don't speak over other people
- Don't swear or make inappropriate comments
- Listen and respect each other
- Be aware of confidentiality – please do not speak about the group outside of the sessions
- Please turn off or put your mobile phone on silent
- Do you have any other rules to add?

How Common is Brain Injury?

Brain injury is the leading cause of death and disability worldwide.

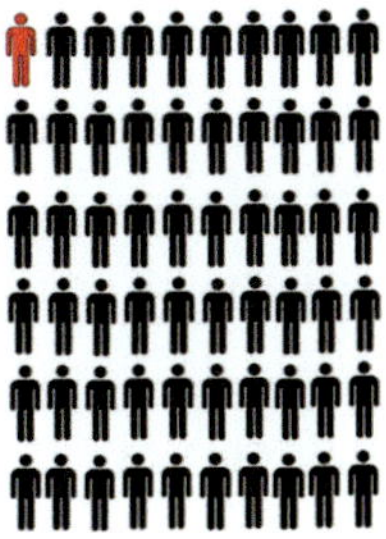

<u>Out of all the people in the UK:</u>

- About **1 in 60** people in the UK go to A&E because of head injuries every year (NICE Guidelines, 2023)
- That means every 90 seconds, someone is admitted to hospital because of an acquired brain injury (Headway, 2018)

<u>Out of these 1 million people:</u>

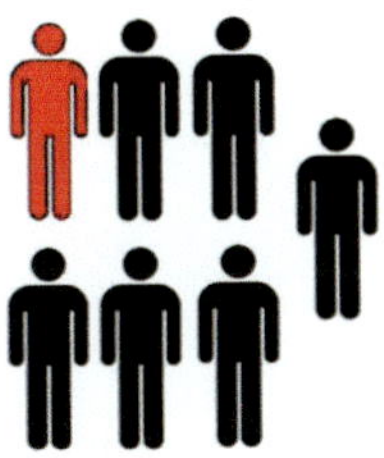

- About **1 in 5** of these people stay in hospital because their injuries are more serious (200,000) (NICE Guidelines, 2023)
- About 40,000 of these have a traumatic brain injury (TBI) (NICE Guidelines, 2023)

<u>Across the UK:</u>

- Approximately 1.3 million people are living with long-term problems because of their brain injury (Headway, 2022)

<u>Other regions across the world:</u>

- In the United States, approximately 1.7 million people sustain new brain injuries every year
- More than 5 million people are living with the long-term effects of brain injury in the US
- An estimated 1.3 million people are living with acquired brain injury in Canada
- Over 160,000 Canadians sustain a brain injury each year
- In the European Union, brain injury accounts for well over 2 million hospitalisations each year, with 1.5 million TBIs resulting in hospitalisation
- In Australia, over 450,000 people, or approximately 1 in 45, live with brain injury

<u>Types of brain injuries:</u>

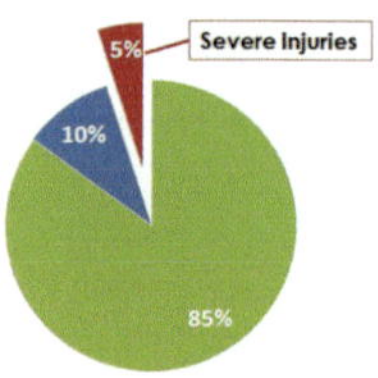

- Minor or mild: about 85% of all brain injuries
- Moderate: about 10% of all brain injuries
- Severe: about 5% of all brain injuries

More men than women have brain injuries.

	The Two Halves of the Brain
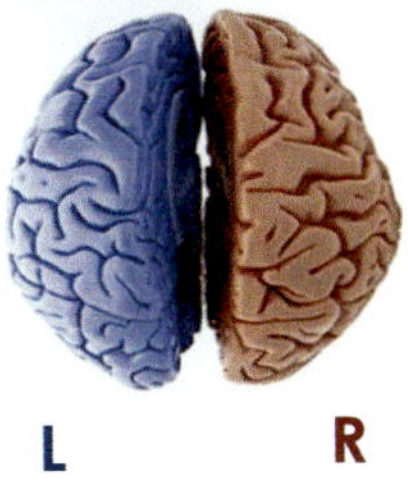	The brain has two halves or 'hemi-spheres'.
	These are called: • The **left** hemisphere, and • The **right** hemisphere
	Movement
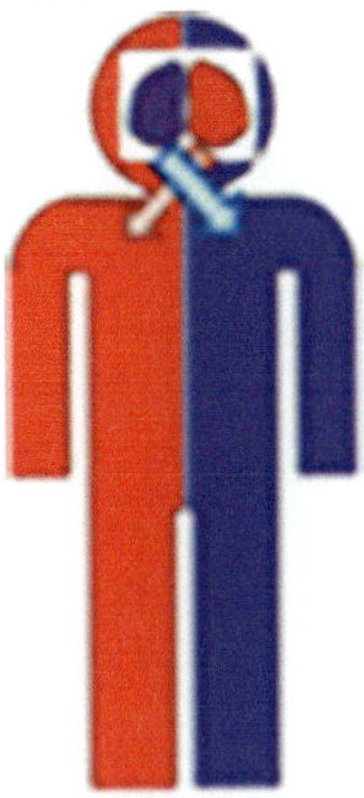	These control the movements of the opposite side of the body: • The **left** hemisphere controls your **right** side, and • The **right** hemisphere controls your **left** side
	Thinking abilities
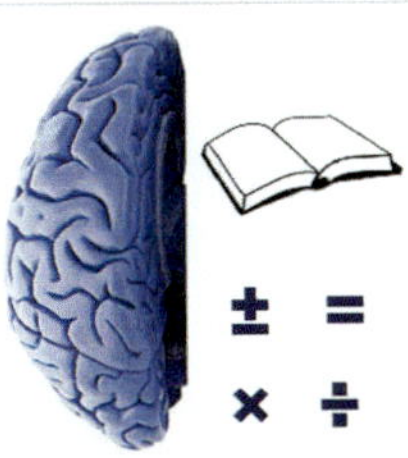	The **left** hemisphere is involved with: • Language (*example*: speaking, reading) • Logical thinking (*example*: maths, rules)
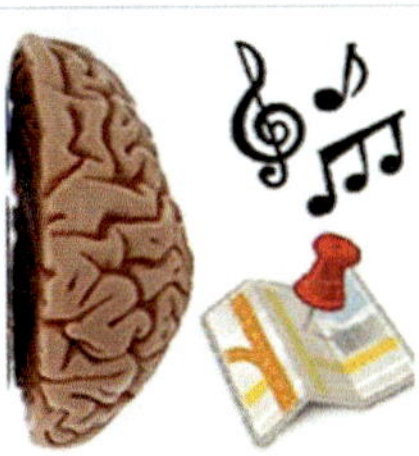	The **right** hemisphere is involved with: • Visual abilities (*example*: drawing, maps) • Music (*example*: singing, speech intonation)

	The Areas of the Brain
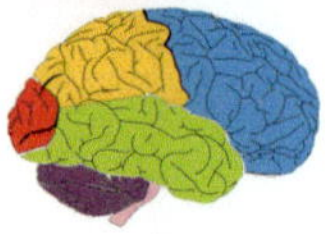	The brain is divided into four main areas called the 'lobes'.
	The **occipital** lobe:
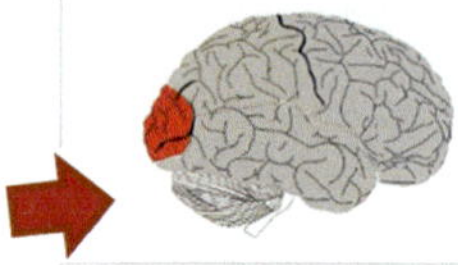	• Vision or sight
	The **parietal** lobe:
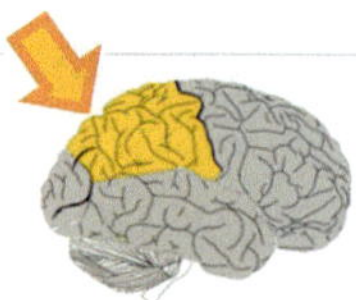	• Touch or sensations
	• Perception and making sense of the world
	The **temporal** lobe:
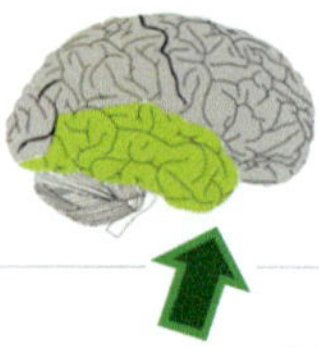	• Memory
	• Language
	The **frontal** lobe:
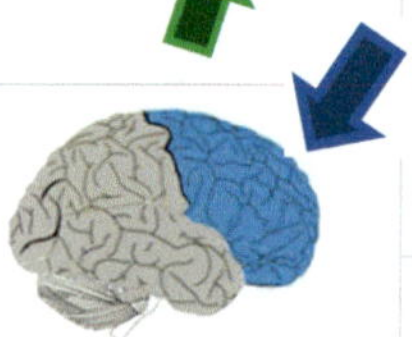	• Executive abilities (organisation, planning)
	• Mood and behaviour ('personality')
	There are two other areas, which are at the base of the brain:
	The **cerebellum**:
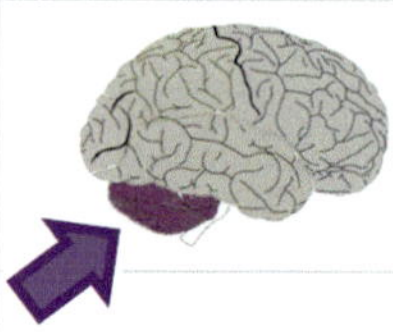	• Balance
	• Coordination of movement
	The **brain stem**
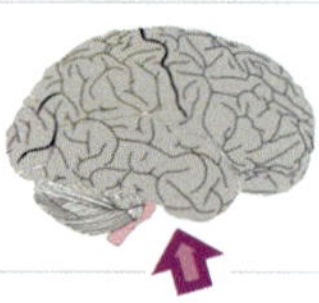	• Vital functions (heartbeat, breathing, blood pressure)

Different Types of Brain Injury

Key fact: The brain needs oxygen to work properly. Oxygen is like the 'fuel of the brain'. Blood carries oxygen around the body and brain in blood vessels. Brain injury is caused when parts of the brain do not get enough blood.

Stroke

A stroke is when blood does not get to a particular part of the brain.

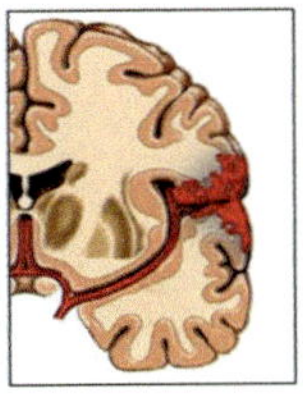

A stroke can happen when:

- A blood vessel gets blocked (ischaemic)
- A blood vessel bursts, and the blood leaks out (haemorrhagic)

Hypoxia

When not enough oxygen gets to the brain, it is called hypoxia. Very severe hypoxia is called anoxia.

This is often caused by heart attacks, but there are many other causes, including poisoning, near-drowning, and suicide attempts.

Traumatic brain injury

The brain can be injured by a blow to the head:

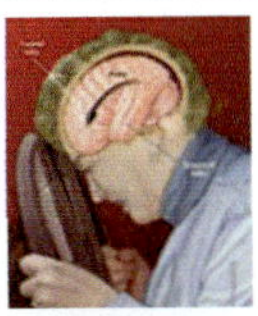

<u>Closed</u> head injury: This is a blow to the outside of the head, such as in a car accident or fall

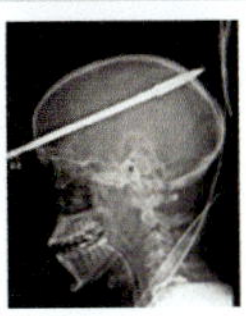

<u>Open</u> head injury: This is when the injury gets into the brain itself – for example, due to a gunshot or piercing injury

	Tumours
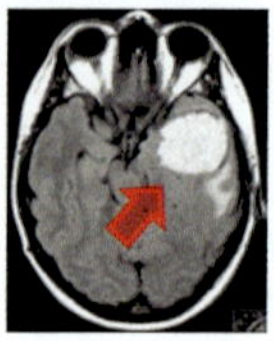	Tumours are when cells grow abnormally. This leads to a mass of extra tissue inside the brain.
	Tumours take up extra space inside the skull and can put pressure on the brain. They are sometimes cancerous.
	Infections
	The brain can become infected; this is called encephalitis

Changes Since ______'s Brain Injury

Since _____ brain injury happened:

Are there any changes that can be seen?

____

____

____

Are there any changes that cannot be seen (such as thinking abilities, behaviours, etc.)?

____

____

____

____

____

____

What positive things have helped since the brain injury?

____

____

____

Session 2

Physical Changes After Brain Injury

	This session includes:	
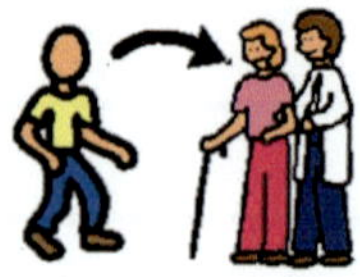		Common physical changes
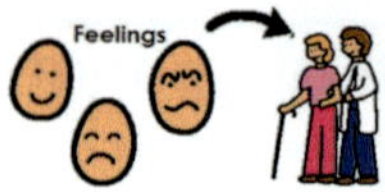		Feelings about physical changes
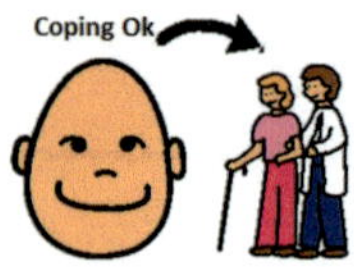		Coping with physical changes

Common Physical Difficulties

Brain injuries can lead to physical problems. These depend on where exactly the brain injury is.

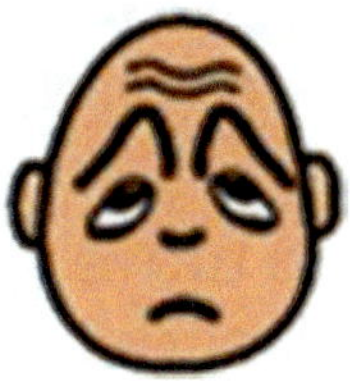

Tiredness

It is common to feel tired more easily after a brain injury.

- Some people find they can't do as much exercise
- Many people need to take more breaks and rests when recovering from a brain injury

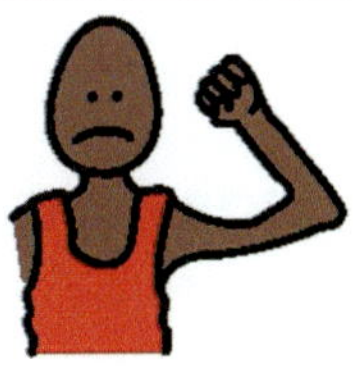

Muscle weakness

After brain injury, it is common to have weakness in muscles (legs, arms, face)

- This is often on one side of the body more than the other.

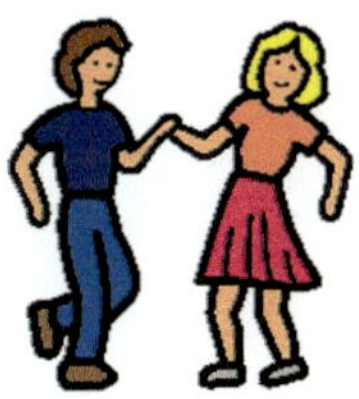

Coordination

It is common for brain injuries to lead to:

- Problems coordinating movements, such as making a cup of tea
- Problems controlling movement, such as difficulties writing or staying still

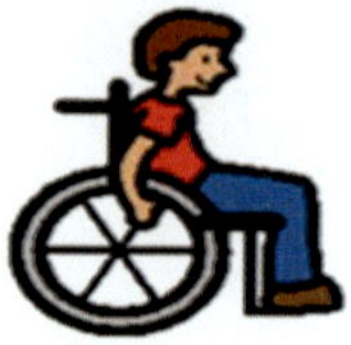	**Walking and movement**
	Many people are less mobile after brain injuries. For example:
	• Some people find it difficult to move at all and need help to roll in bed or sit up
	• Some people are able to move but find it difficult to walk or get up from a chair
	Increased muscle tone
	This is when muscles are tense and difficult to relax
	• It can make it difficult to stretch muscles
	• It can be very painful
	There can be physical changes in a healthy loved one's life too
	These can include:
	• Impaired sleep
	• Changes in appetite
	• Inability to exercise
	• Increased tiredness

Feelings About Physical Changes

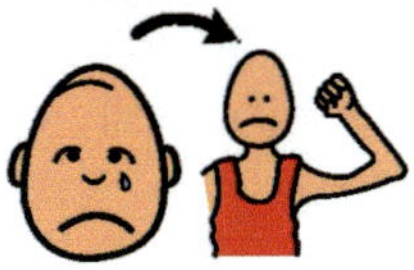

It is common to feel upset about your loved one's physical changes and how they are affecting your life. Here are some common feelings.

Frustration

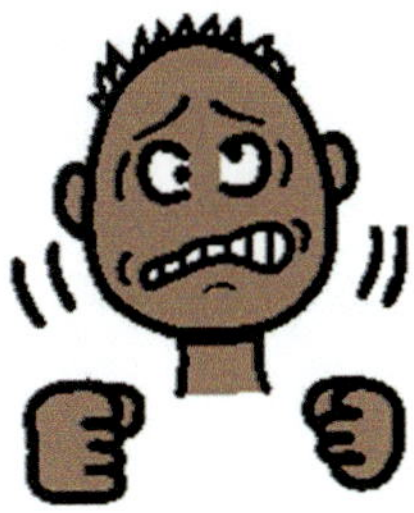

When people cannot do as much, this can lead to frustration. Some things that can cause this are when your loved one needs:

- Assistance with getting out of bed
- Help with going to the toilet
- Help with mobility throughout the day

Anger

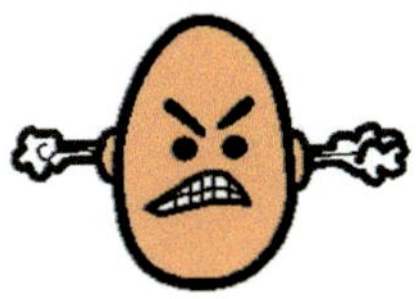

Some people can feel angry about their loved one's physical problems:

- You might be angry at the world or angry at God because of the brain injury
- You might become angry with the people around you, such as family, friends, or the one you're caring for

Sadness

Realising a loved one cannot do as much as they used to can lead people to feel sad or low:

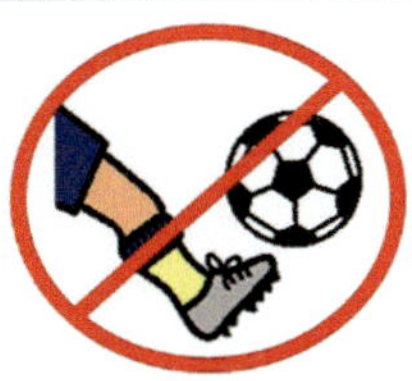

- You may focus on things you can no longer do, such as walking or playing sport
- This can make you feel very low and not want to do much at all

	Worry and anxiety
	You might find yourself worrying more often about your loved one's physical abilities, especially if they might fall and injure themselves further.
	Deny problems or feel numb
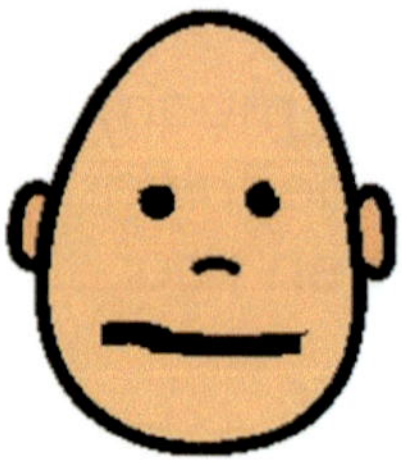	Some people find it very difficult to think about the problems they have and all the life changes this will lead to:
	• You might try not to think about these, or 'play them down'
	• You might feel overwhelmed and unable to think about your loved one's problems
	• You might deny the fact that these are long-lasting issues and so refuse the help offered

	Coping with Physical Changes
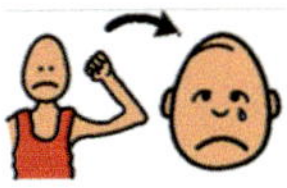	Physical problems after brain injury are common and can make people feel upset. However, people often cope well with these.
	Here are some things people find to help them cope.
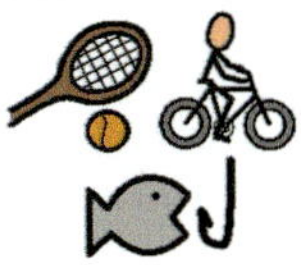	**Do things you enjoy!**
	It is important to keep doing things that you enjoy – for example:
	• Listening to music, watching television, or reading
	• Spending time with other people, such as friends and family
	Find other ways to do it!
	If physical problems are holding your loved one back, it can help to find other ways for them to do what they want.
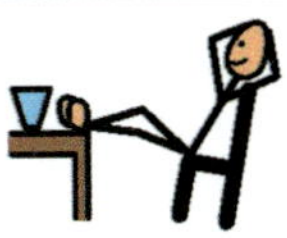	• They can try taking more breaks and taking more time to do a task
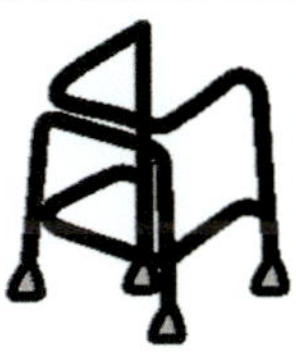	• They can use equipment to help – for example, a walking aid or wheelchair so you and your loved one can still go out
	Sometimes, you won't be able to physically do the activities you used to enjoy due to caring responsibilities. When this is the case, are there other ways of achieving the same goal?

	• For example if you can't go to the gym, can you find another way to exercise while remaining at home for your loved one?
	Ask other people for support!
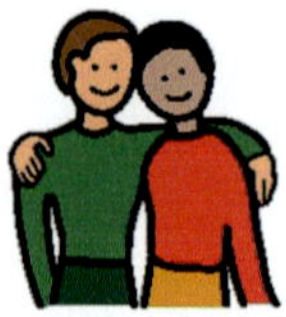	Sometimes physical problems mean we cannot do something by ourselves, and so we need to ask for help.
	Lean on friends, family, and professionals for support.

Session 3

Mental Process Changes After Brain Injury
(cognitive thinking styles, mood and behaviour)

	This session includes:	
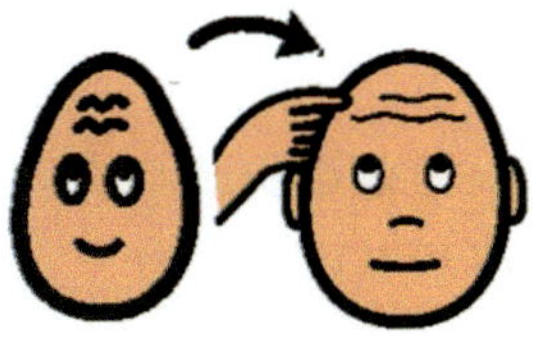		Common mental process changes
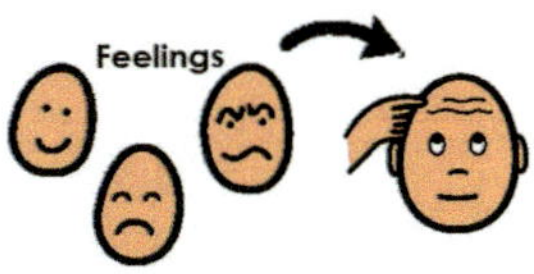		Feelings about mental process changes
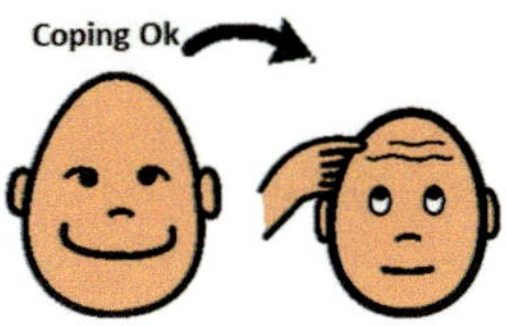		Coping with mental process changes

	Common Thinking (Cognitive) Difficulties
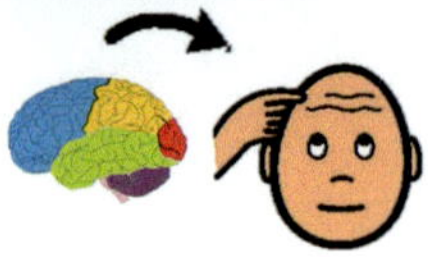	The brain is responsible for our thinking abilities. These are also called 'cognitive abilities'.
	Brain injuries can lead to cognitive problems.
	Again, the exact problems depend on where the brain is damaged. Everyone is different.
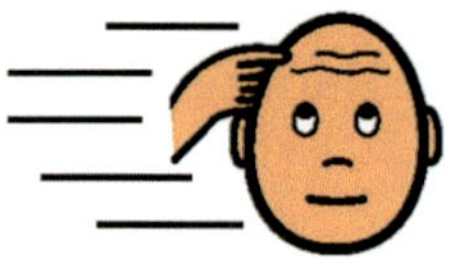	**Slower thinking speed**
	This is called reduced 'processing speed', meaning that it takes longer to take on board and make sense of information.
	This is very common after brain injuries.
	Difficulties this may lead to in daily life include:
	• Not being able to keep up with other people's conversations
	• Taking longer to do something compared to before the brain injury
	• Not taking all the information in, so that not all the information can be learned
	Memory
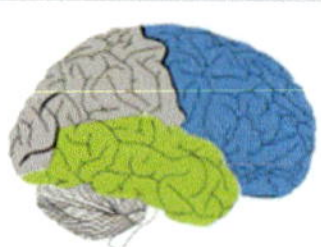	Memory problems are especially linked with injuries in the **frontal** and **temporal** lobes.

	Memory problems can affect:
	• Recently learned information
	• Older information
	• Remembering to do something in the future
	Memories come in two main types:
	• Explicit memories: Information people have conscious access to
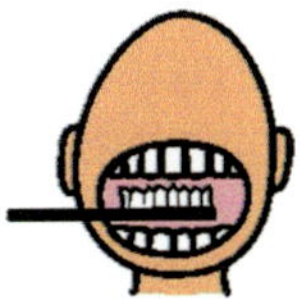	• Implicit memories: Knowledge people do not need to consciously access (such as how to brush teeth)
	This means that, sometimes, people with brain injuries can carry on doing daily tasks, but they find it difficult to adapt to new situations and learn new information.
	'Executive' abilities
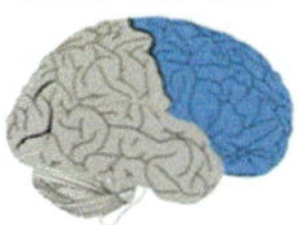	Solving new problems involves a lot of different thinking abilities, most of which are in the **frontal** lobes.
	These are referred to as 'executive functions', because they are like a company's executive board, which oversees all the other abilities
	Some examples of executive abilities include:
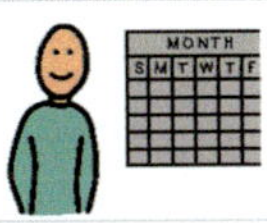	• Planning before and during tasks
	• Organising things
	• Solving problems that come up
	• Starting actions at the right time

	• Stopping actions when needed
	• Dividing attention between different tasks
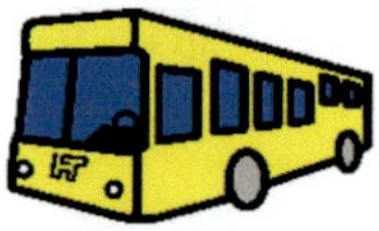	A good example is planning a journey by public transport, as people use most of these abilities to do this.
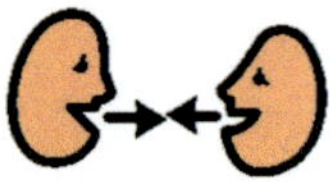	**Language**
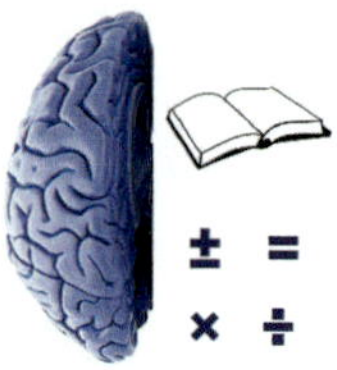	The **left** hemisphere is most important for language, but **right** hemisphere damage can cause subtle difficulties (for example, the 'music' or tone of speech).
	These include people making themselves understood (expressive) and understanding other people (receptive).
	Making themselves understood includes:
	• Speaking (words and grammar)
	• Writing
	• Non-verbal speech (tone of voice, speed)
	• Non-verbal communication (body language)
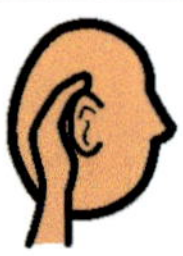	Understanding other people includes:
	• Understanding speech
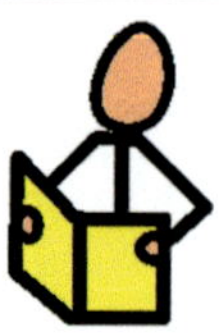	• Reading
	• Making sense of what people mean even when they don't say it (social inferencing)

	Awareness of difficulties
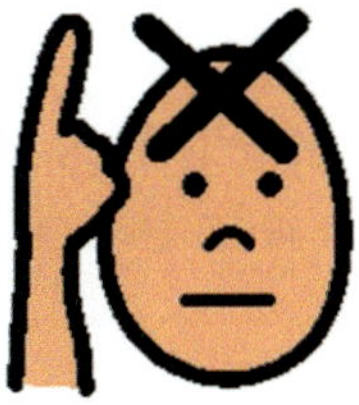	The brain is also important for people to make sense of what has happened to them.
	Sometimes, brain injury can cause problems with being aware of new difficulties.
	This lack of awareness is normally a mix of:
	• Changes in the brain because of brain injury
	• Avoiding thoughts about difficulties
	This is very important. If people do not understand that they have problems, it can be difficult for them to find solutions to these problems.
	People who have difficulties with awareness can:
	• Say that they don't have any problems at all
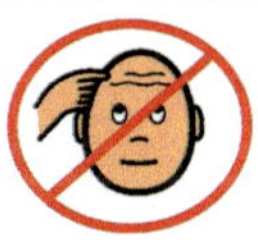	• Report some problems, such as physical changes, but not others, such as thinking changes
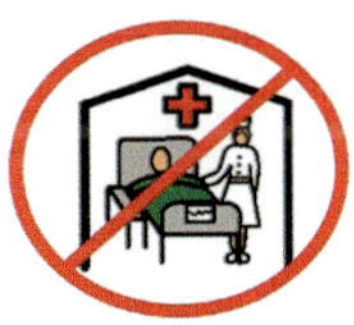	• Feel like they can get back to everyday life
	• Feel like they should not have to work with rehabilitation therapists

	Common Mood and Behavioural Difficulties
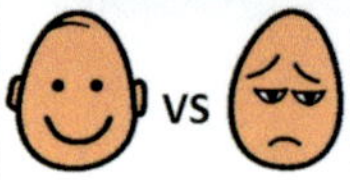	The brain controls our mood and behaviour. Injury can lead to difficulties depending on where the brain is injured.
	Rapid changes in mood
	Some people find that their mood changes more rapidly:
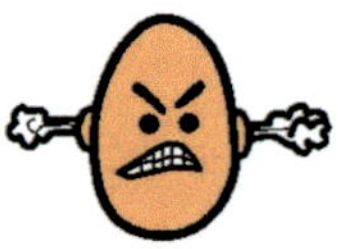	• They become angry very quickly and find it difficult to control or manage their temper
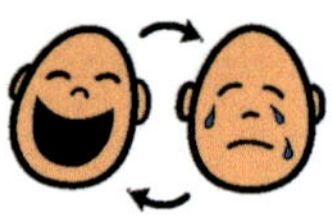	• They may find that their mood changes rapidly, crying or laughing suddenly.
	Sadness
	Many people find themselves feeling low or depressed. This can be quite normal but can also lead to feelings of demotivation and apathy.
	Anxiety
	There may be an increase in worries after a brain injury and these can interfere with the rehabilitation process.
	Acting impulsively
	Many people behave or think impulsively after brain injury.
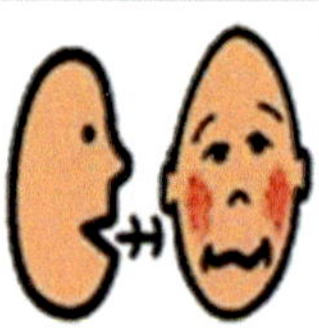	• <u>Inappropriate behaviour</u>: Acting without thinking can make other people uncomfortable or embarrassed – for example, making a sexual comment to someone.

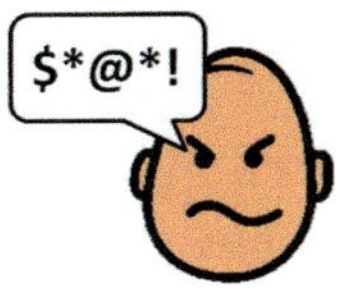	• <u>Foul language</u>: When people are impulsive they can be rude or abusive. They may use profanities and swear more than they would have beforehand or make cruel, out-of-character comments.
	Repeated behaviour
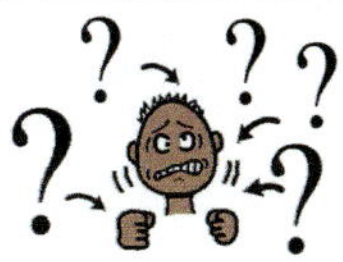	After brain injury, people can get stuck on some actions or thoughts more easily. This can be due to brain changes or attempts to feel calmer.
	• People may ask the same questions over and over again, or say the same things
	• People can get stuck on certain thoughts, e.g., someone stealing from them

	Feelings About Cognitive Changes
	Cognitive, mood and behavioural problems will have a big impact on people's lives; these can be very frustrating at times.
	It is common to feel upset about these changes. However, everyone reacts in their own way.
	Here are some of these common feelings:
	Confusion
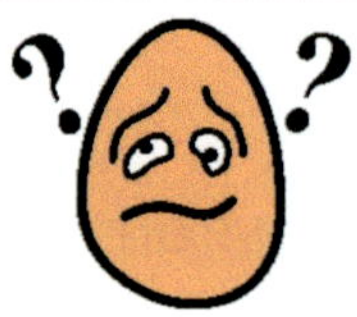	Difficulties with thinking abilities can make your loved one seem very different; and this, in turn, can make your relationship feel confusing.
	• You may need to take on more of a caring role than you did before the brain injury – this can affect your identity within the relationship
	• You may be struggling to understand what has happened to your loved one, especially the medical aspect and what their recovery trajectory is likely to be
	Worry and anxiety
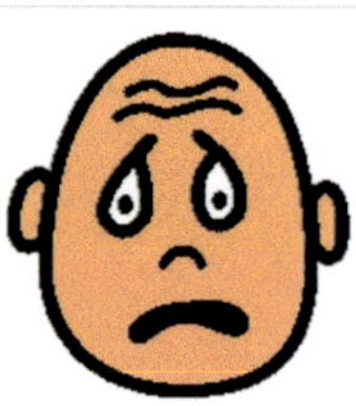	If your loved one is experiencing cognitive difficulties, this can make it difficult for them to make sense of the world or predict what will happen. This uncertainty and doubt often lead to anxiety for both them and yourself.

	• You may worry about their safety at home unless they are constantly supervised, as they may forget they cannot do what they used to
	• You may worry about how they will manage independently, when it is difficult for them to carry out day-to-day tasks
	Frustration and anger
	Cognitive difficulties can be very frustrating. For example:
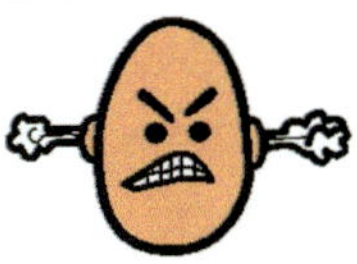	• You may get frustrated and angry because your loved one is slower with their thinking
	• You may find it difficult to communicate things that you need from your loved one as they don't seem to understand
	Sadness
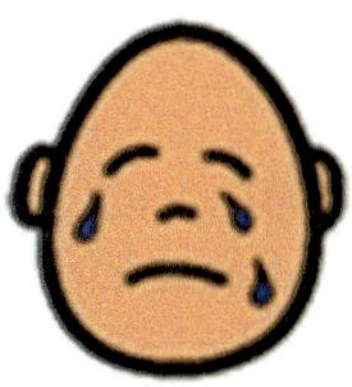	Cognitive problems can lead people to feel low, often because they're aware of the things they can no longer do with their loved ones – such as having in-depth conversations, enjoying books or films together, or going on excursions.

	Feelings About Mood Changes
	Mood and behaviour changes have a big impact on your lives.
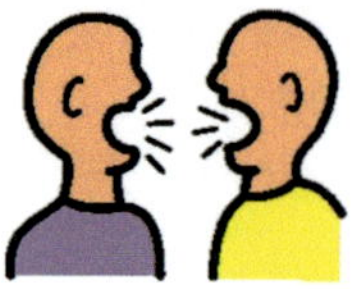	These changes often cause difficulties with other people, which in turn can result in you feeling upset or that you can no longer enjoy the company of others.
	Here are some common feelings:
	Confusion
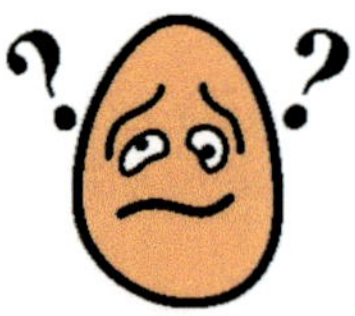	Often other people will act differently with you because of changes in how your loved one behaves. These changes in how others act can be confusing.
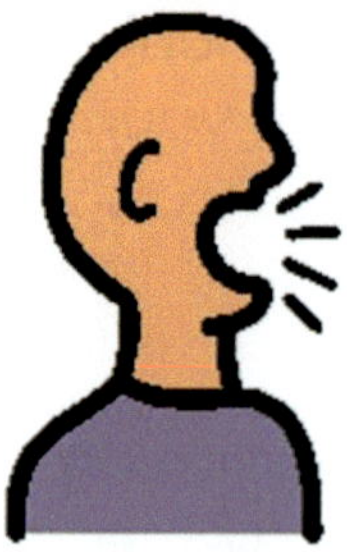	• If your loved one loses their temper more easily, this can make other people feel scared or upset, and so they might also avoid you
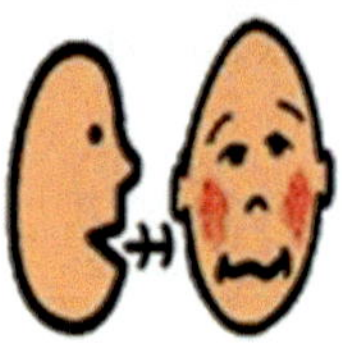	• If your loved one is more blunt and says what they think without thinking through the consequences, this can make others feel uncomfortable and may even result in friends no longer wanting to visit. • This can leave you feeling confused that they no longer want to see you when you need all the support you can get!

	Anxiety
	Brain injury to a loved one can make us feel more vulnerable and worried.
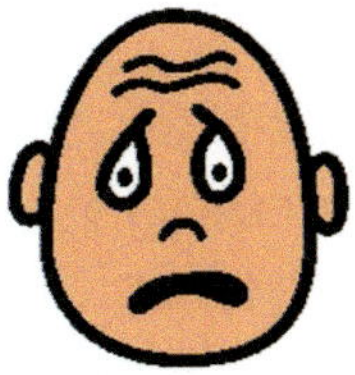	• Feelings and worries can seem stronger and more difficult to manage after a loved one's brain injury
	• It can be more difficult to feel reassured by others
	• We can catastrophise more easily, allowing our thoughts to go to the worst-case scenario more often
	Frustration and anger
	Difficulties with mood and behaviour can make you feel angry or frustrated with your loved one or yourself.
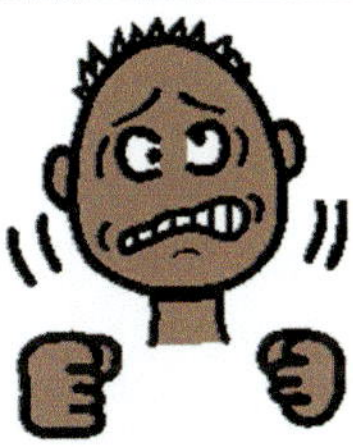	• When you find it difficult to stop yourself from doing something that is not helpful (like losing your temper), it can be frustrating
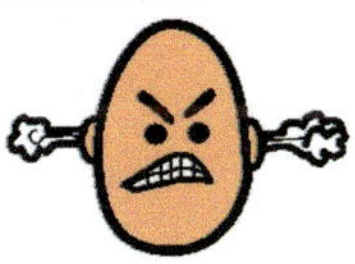	• You can become angry at other people when they act differently towards you or your loved one – for example, if they seem to be uncomfortable
	Feeling misunderstood or not valued
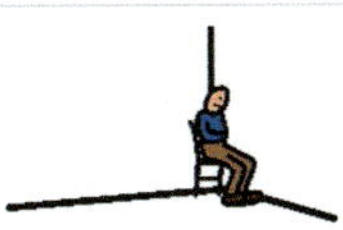	When other people act differently towards you, you can feel like they do not care or are not listening. This may lead to you behaving differently as well:

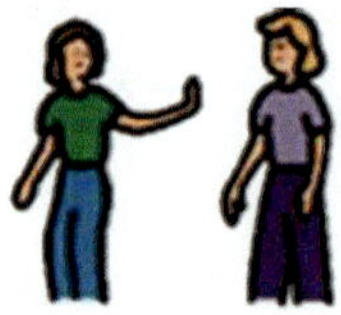	• Shouting and getting angry when others do not understand that your life has been turned upside down
	• Friends may distance themselves, as they do not know how to manage your loved one's changes (especially cognitive and behavioural changes) – this may lead to feelings of not being valued any more

Coping with Cognitive Changes

Cognitive problems after brain injury are common. They affect those who are caring for the individual as much as the individual themselves. Below are some practical suggestions to help:

Use strategies

There are many skills the person with the brain injury can learn to help overcome cognitive difficulties:

- Memory problems: Try memory strategies, e.g., anagrams, making stories out of information or picturing things, using memory aids such as diaries, alarms on mobile phones, calendars

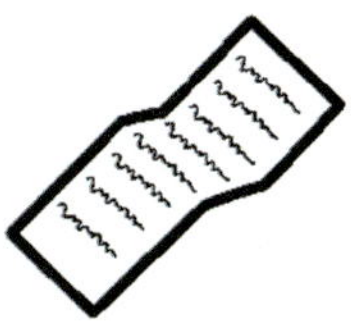

- Poor organisation: Learn skills to break tasks down into small steps, with checklists to keep on track

Use supports and gadgets

Many people have some memory and organisation difficulties. This means that everyone can benefit from helpful strategies.

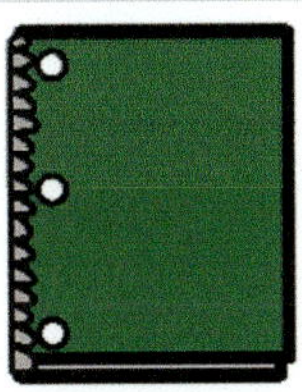

There are many pieces of equipment available that you can use to help with cognitive difficulties:

- Simple aids: Notebooks and calendars

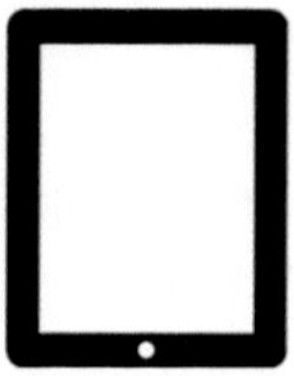 iPad	• Gadgets: Electronic organisers (mobile phones, iPads) and alarms
	Ask other people for support
	Sometimes it can be difficult to manage new tasks:
	• Ask the **psychologist** or **occupational therapist** for help with memory or organisation
	• Ask the **speech and language therapist** for help with language and communication problems

	Coping with Mood Changes
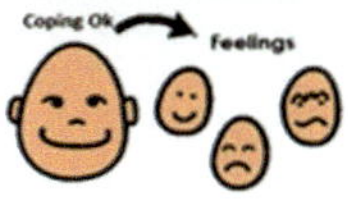	Mood and behaviour changes after brain injury are common; however, people can often cope well with these.
	Here are some things people find that help them cope:
	Do things you enjoy!
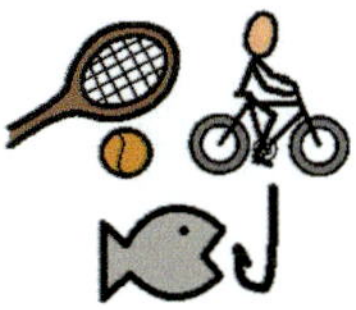	Feeling happier with their life in general can help your loved one stay calm and manage their emotions. For example:
	• Listening to music or watching television
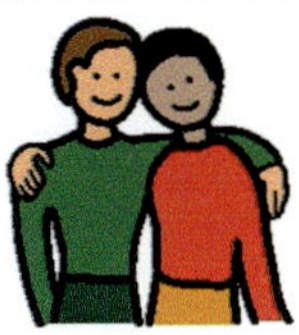	• Spending time with other people, e.g., friends and family
	Use strategies
	There are many skills your loved one can learn to help them manage their emotions and behaviour:
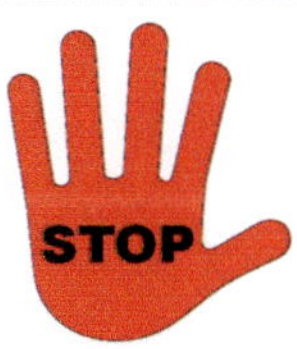	• When they start getting angry, teach them to **stop** and give themselves time to calm down
	• When they feel vulnerable and uncertain, write down information that is comforting

	Ask other people for support
	It might help if other people know your loved one has a brain injury. This helps them make sense of your loved one's mood and behaviour changes. It is also useful to ask for help:
	• If your loved one is feeling upset or angry
	• If your loved one is confused about the way other people are treating them

	Strategies to Help with Your Own Emotions
	Brain injury to a loved one can leave us with many emotions. You need strategies to help you cope with these emotions as well as strategies to help with your loved one's disabilities. These can come in three forms: problem-focused, emotion-focused, or distraction-focused.
	Problem-focused: • Read up on brain injury • Teach loved ones to use gadgets • Help loved ones with their rehabilitation tasks • Set alarms as reminders
	Emotion-focused: • Go to a support group • Talk to friends • Have a good cry • Use faith to help
	Distraction-focused: • Go for a walk • Read a book • Watch TV/film • Listen to music • Do something creative

Session 4

Lifestyle Changes After Brain Injury

	This session includes:	
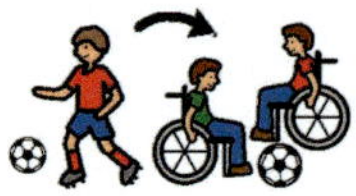		Lifestyle changes after brain injury
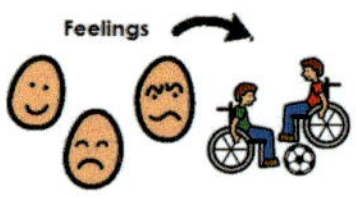		Feelings about lifestyle changes
 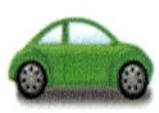		Coping with lifestyle changes

	Lifestyle Changes After Brain Injury
	Reclaiming your life
	Some people find that their lifestyle is different once their loved one has left rehabilitation.
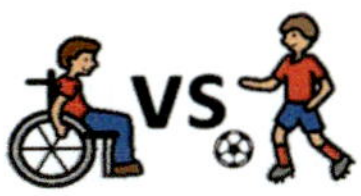	Most of the time, this means that there are things that need to change about how you and your loved one live your lives.
	Some common differences are:
	Structure: It can help both you and your loved one to keep to a structure so that each day can be more predictable
	Socialising: Keeping in contact with friends and family is important for both you and your loved one, although this may be challenging at times
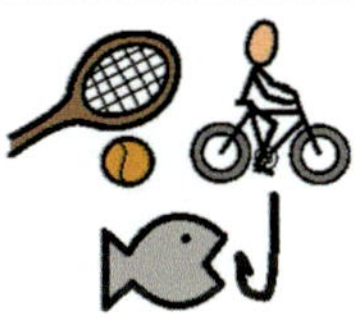	Work and hobbies: Many individuals want to go back to work, but are unable to due to their brain injury; equally you may find that the additional caring responsibilities that you now have make returning to employment more difficult, if not impossible. This is also the case for many hobbies – for example, going to the gym, exercising, playing instruments. These can all seem more difficult when you have a caring role at home.

	<u>Role changes</u>: Since the brain injury, the role you used to have will often have changed to that of a carer rather than a wife, husband, child, parent, etc. This may be difficult, and you may benefit from talking therapy. In some cases, you may now need to provide the sole income to the family. You may also need to take on board more of the household or driving responsibilities than was the case before the brain injury. If it is your partner who has had the brain injury, then there may be a change in your intimacy, which can be difficult for both of you.

	Feelings About Lifestyle Changes
	Lifestyle changes will have a big impact on people's lives, and this can stir up strong feelings.
	They can be worried about the future, or have strong feelings about the changes they will have to make.
	Here are some common feelings.
	Anxiety and worry
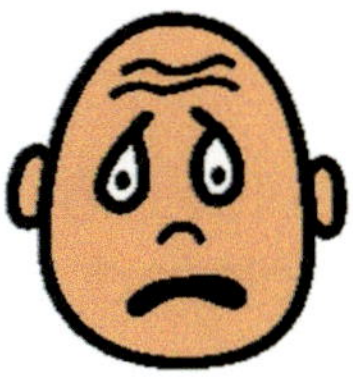	Many people say that they are looking forward to getting back to their lives, once their loved one is out of hospital or rehabilitation, but they also feel worried about the way things have changed. They may have:
	• Worries about how their loved one will manage in their home with the challenges the brain injury may have caused (stairs, difficulties in the kitchen, personal care, etc.)
	• Worries about how their loved one will fit into their previous social circle
	• Worries about how well their loved one will be able to do the things they used to do, e.g., work.
	These worries are understandable and are normal. With the right support, most people manage.

	Feeling down
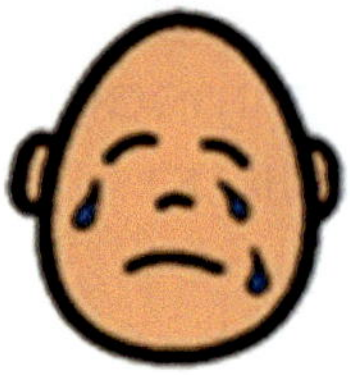	Some people really look forward to having their loved one home but then they find some things more difficult, which can make them feel sad or down.
	It is helpful to remember that there are many ways to continue doing the things you find important, and the things that you enjoy, with good support and some changes.
	Feeling isolated and helpless
	It is normal to feel helpless in the face of brain injury. Many people feel isolated at this difficult time, especially as they often do not know others who have been through the process of having a loved one acquire a brain injury. Support groups such as those provided by Headway or the Stroke Association can really help with this feeling of isolation
	Feeling shocked, frightened, and having a sense of 'Why me?'
	Again, these are normal emotions to feel, especially in the early stages of recovery from a brain injury for both yourselves and your loved ones. It can help to talk to professionals about the reasons for and likely prognosis of the brain injury. But it is a good idea not to Google everything, as this can make the future look very bleak! Rather, take each day as it comes.

	Coping with Lifestyle Changes
	While your loved one is at home, many people can help them on their path to recovery.
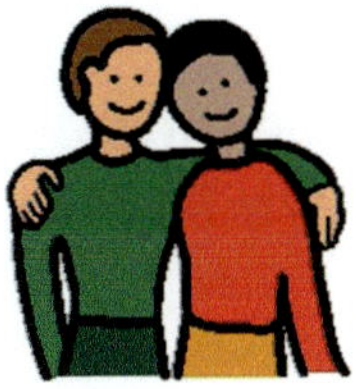	**Family and friends**
	Having the support of your family and your friends can be very helpful for both yourself and your loved one:
	• They can help with practical things, such as checking both you and your loved one are doing all right with everyday tasks, now that your loved one is home
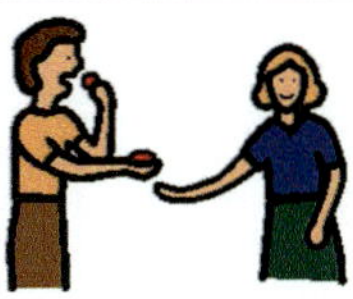	• They can give emotional support, and the chance for both of you to talk safely about any difficulties that have arisen since your loved one returned home
	Health services
NHS	Once you leave rehabilitation, you can still access health services in your local area. For example:
	• Your GP
	• Community therapists
	Social services
Lewisham	Social services will help you to get the care you need for your loved one. For some people, this might be:

	• Arranging a suitable place for you to live
	• A care package which pays for carers to visit you at home
	Charities and support groups
	Headway is a group that works to improve life after brain injury. Some of the helpful things they do are the provision of:
	• Support groups
	• Vocational rehabilitation

References

Headway – the Brain Injury Association. (2018). *Acquired brain injury – The numbers behind the hidden disability*. https://www.headway.org.uk/media/7866/brain-injury-statistics-methodology-injury-categories-and-further-notes-2018.pdf.

Headway – the Brain Injury Association. (2022). *Acquired brain injury & the criminal justice system: A briefing for probation staff*. https://www.headway.org.uk/media/9917/acquired-brain-injury-and-the-criminal-justice-system-briefing-for-probation-staff.pdf.

National Institute for Health and Care Excellence. (2023). *Head injury: Assessment and early management*. https://www.nice.org.uk/guidance/ng232.

With thanks to:

Dr Kevin Tierney, clinical psychologist

Index